NATURAL
SECRETS
DRUG COMPANIES
DON'T WANT YOU TO KNOW ABOUT

NATURAL
SECRETS
DRUG COMPANIES
DON'T WANT YOU TO KNOW ABOUT

THE STRAIGHT TRUTH
ABOUT NUTRITION, DISEASE,
& NATURAL CURES

MARK A. STEVENS
WITH CHRISTINE JONES

TATE PUBLISHING & Enterprises

This title is also available as a Tate Out Loud product. Visit www.tatepublishing.com for more information.

Published by Tate Publishing & Enterprises, LLC
127 E. Trade Center Terrace | Mustang, Oklahoma 73064 USA
1.888.361.9473 | www.tatepublishing.com

Tate Publishing is committed to excellence in the publishing industry. The company reflects the philosophy established by the founders, based on Psalm 68:11,
"The Lord gave the word and great was the company of those who published it."

Book design copyright © 2008 by Tate Publishing, LLC. All rights reserved.
Cover design by Kandi Evans
Interior design by Jacob Crissup

Published in the United States of America

ISBN: 978-1-60604-286-1
1. Health and Fitness: Nutrition
2. Medical: Drug Guides
08.07.16

DEDICATION

This book is lovingly dedicated to my mother, Georgia, whose determined spirit in the face of daunting health challenges set my feet upon the path toward a lifelong passion for discovering the secrets of naturally vibrant, good health.

Mark A. Stevens

TABLE OF CONTENTS

CHAPTER ONE
The Billion-Dollar Business of Illness

Prescription-Drug Mania

In today's fast-paced culture, it is becoming increasingly difficult to maintain optimum good health—physically, mentally, and emotionally. We rise each morning, after too little recuperative sleep, feeling drained before the day even begins. We feed our bodies the empty calories of fast food or skip meals entirely. Arriving home at the end of a stressful day, we fall into our comfortable recliners with absolutely no thought of healthful exercise. Sound familiar? This is the daily pattern of the majority of Americans today, and quite honestly, it's killing us. Heart disease is at an all-time high, as is obesity, high cholesterol, diabetes, and a myriad of other debilitating health issues.

Literally millions of people in the United States alone take some sort of prescription every day. This prescription-loving environment seems to have embraced the attitude of "Have a problem? Take a pill." Too little thought is given to maintaining proper health habits, resulting in too much dependence on synthetic chemicals promising to cure all our ills. The terrifying truth, however, is that prescription drugs often simply mask the underlying symptoms of our bodies crying out for the proper nutrition, exercise, and rest that they require for optimum health.

Many doctors exacerbate this problem by recommending prescription drugs as the single viable solution rather than educating their patients on the hazards and disastrous effects of poor diet choices and sedentary lifestyles. Shockingly, even the most prestigious medical schools place the cause and affects of nutrition in the human body at the very bottom of their curriculums, with doctors frequently taking only one course in nutrition during their entire scholastic experience.

This prescription mania is further fueled by mammoth pharmaceutical companies. These goliath drug manufacturers offer doctors and their staffs everything from unlimited samples to free meals to luxurious, all-expense-paid vacations. The business of prescription drugs is a highly lucrative one with extremely high stakes, as evidenced by the billions of prescriptions being written every year.

But if prescription drugs are the solution, then why is America increasingly filled with sick, overweight, depressed citizens? Why do we rank so abysmally low in health and longevity compared to other industrialized nations?

The Unseen Danger

The Food and Drug Administration, also known

as the FDA, is responsible for the regulation of prescription drugs. This responsibility includes thorough investigation and verification of the safety of any new prescription drug before it is placed on the market for public consumption. So with such reassuring regulations in place to verify the quality and safety of our medicines, should we be worried about unsafe drugs entering the marketplace? The overwhelming answer is yes. Thousands upon thousands of people are seriously injured each year by dangerous and unexpected side effects of prescription drugs. And even worse, over 100,000 deaths each year are attributed to the negative effects of drugs. Keep in mind that these heart-wrenching tragedies occur in spite of all the FDA regulations in place.

This problem has become so widespread that a well-known consumer health advocate and outspoken critic of pharmaceutical companies has been quoted as saying that the drug industry is freely killing Americans. This health advocate went on to say, "The entire drug industry, including the monopolistic drug giants and their FDA co-conspirator, has clearly become the single greatest threat to the health and safety of the American people. And yet the FDA continues to push more drugs onto more Americans than ever before, all while pretending these drugs are safe and effective when, in reality, they are neither." (1)

These dangerous drugs can include both prescription and over-the-counter medicines that consumers take to improve their health and quality of life. However, many medications have such serious adverse effects that, when weighed against their benefits, they are actually more harmful than helpful. The injuries caused by long-term exposure to some prescription drugs are often permanent and life threatening. These injuries can include birth defects; damage to organs such as the heart, liver, or kidneys; damage to the brain or nervous system; and many types of cancer.

For example, Prempro and other hormone replacement therapy drugs can cause pulmonary embolism, strokes, and deep-vein thrombosis in some women. In July 2002, a federal study released findings that long-term use of Prempro leads to a significantly increased risk of breast cancer, heart disease, and stroke. This study, called the Women's Health Initiative (WHI), revealed that virtually everything the pharmaceutical companies had been telling doctors and their patients about the benefits and risks of Prempro was dead wrong. The study concluded that the risks of Prempro vastly outweighed its benefits and urged women to stop taking the drug immediately. Many other studies followed, finding similar and sometimes even more alarming results.

Wyeth, the manufacturer of Prempro, scrambled to change its warning label, but for thousands of women it was too late. Breast cancer had already developed, and their lives had been forever changed. In the years since the introduction of prescription hormone replacement therapy drugs like Prempro, a breast cancer epidemic has been created.

Vioxx was touted as the next miracle drug for pain relief when it was introduced in 1999. Doctors had prescribed Vioxx to over two million people when its manufacturer, Merck & Company, withdrew the drug from the worldwide market in 2004 after a three-year trial revealed that the use of Vioxx led to a fifty percent greater chance of heart attack, stroke, blood clots, and even death.[2] The FDA estimates the prescription drug Vioxx may have caused up to 140,000 cases of serious heart disease since 1999.

Accutane is the brand name for isotretinion, a drug prescribed for acne. Accutane came under the scrutiny of the FDA largely due to its link to birth defects. Yet more recently, the drug manufacturer's failure to perform adequate clinical trials to evaluate a possible link between Accutane and suicide attempts has come to light.

According to FDA reports, Accutane may

cause depression, psychosis, suicide attempts, and suicide. However, discontinuing Accutane therapy may not be sufficient to stop these effects. Feelings of depression may be episodic upon discontinuing use of this prescription drug, but patients report suffering ongoing feelings of loneliness, sadness, chronic loss of energy, irritability, and changes in sleep patterns.

OxyContin was approved by the FDA in 1996 as a twelve-hour time-release pain medication for the treatment of moderate to severe chronic pain experienced by patients with terminal cancer, paralysis, and musculoskeletal conditions. The advantage of OxyContin over other pain medications is that the pills are required once every twelve hours rather than every three to six as required with alternative pain medications.

However, a myriad of frightening problems stem from this painkiller. If the tablets are broken, chewed, or crushed, the patient can absorb a potentially fatal dose as it is rapidly released in the bloodstream.

OxyContin has further received the reputation as a drug more addictive than heroin. It is no surprise, then, that as a popular black market drug, OxyContin tends to be consumed improperly by addicts. This drug has been linked to thousands of overdose deaths nationwide, and the death rate is expected to increase as its popularity on the black market grows.

With heart disease at an all-time high, we have become increasingly aware of the need to reduce harmful cholesterol levels. However, many cholesterol-lowering drugs such as Crestor have serious side effects. Crestor reduces cholesterol levels by blocking the liver from producing bad cholesterol (LDL). This prescription drug became the sixth cholesterol-lowering statin drug on the U.S. market, following drugs like Lipitor, Pravachol, Zocor, and Bacol. However, only three months after its approval, patients who were taking the recommended dosage of Crestor began developing alarming side effects, including kidney failure and muscle damage.

It is important to note that Baycol, another statin drug, has been withdrawn from the market after it was found to cause irreversible kidney damage (rhabdomyolysis).

The drugs mentioned above are not the only threats to health and life posed by pharmaceutical products. Rather, they are simply the tip of a massive iceberg of human misery, debilitation, and death—all in the name of seeking fast, easy chemical solutions to our health issues.

Here is a brief listing of other prescription drugs that are known to have potentially serious, even deadly, consequences:

Actiq: a highly addictive narcotic that has proven fatal consequences

Ketek: a bronchitis drug that causes liver damage and even death

Trasylol: a drug frequently administered prior to heart-bypass surgery known to double the risk of kidney failure and stroke

Ortho Evra: a popular contraceptive patch

known to cause blood clots, heart attack, stroke, and breast cancer

Zyprexa: a schizophrenia medication known to cause diabetes, hyperglycemia, and other blood-sugar disorders

Celebrex: a very popular arthritis medication known to more than double the risk of heart attack and associated cardiovascular problems

Bextra: previously a popular arthritis medication now removed from the market due to significantly increased risk of heart attack, stroke, and other cardiovascular events

Tegison and Soriatane: drugs commonly prescribed for psoriasis that can be extremely harmful to pregnant women and their unborn children

Captopril and Enalopril: high blood-pressure medications known to cause fetal kidney damage and even death when taken during pregnancy

Of course, many prescription drugs have saved lives and improved the quality of life for many, and continue to do so. The issue then becomes taking responsibility for our bodies and our health. Do not make the mistake of being a passive bystander when it comes to your health. Become proactive, do research, and ask questions. For example, are there equally effective natural alternatives that do not present the risk of side effects? Would a change in diet and exercise pattern alleviate the need for a prescription drug? Would high-quality nutritional supplements resolve or relieve the health issue without introducing potentially harmful chemicals into your body? These are extremely valid questions; you owe it to yourself to address them before filling your next prescription.

Doctor and Medication Errors Are Killing Us

According to an article appearing in the *Journal of American Medicine*[3], the most widely circulated medical journal in the world, physician and medication errors are the third leading cause of death in the United States. Yes, you read that right—the third leading killer in the United States, surpassed only by deaths caused by heart disease and cancer.

Keep in mind that this publication chose to fall on the side of caution, deriving its data from studies only involving hospitalized patients. Also, the data used includes deaths only and does not include negative effects resulting in disability or discomfort.

The findings of this report revealed the following shocking figures:

12,000 patients die each year due to unnecessary surgery

7,000 patients die each year due to medication errors by hospital staff

20,000 patients die per year because of other hospital errors

80,000 patients die every year due to infections contracted while hospitalized

> 106,000 patients tragically and needlessly die each year due to negative effects of drugs, even though the drugs were properly administered

Remember, these figures are representative of hospitalized patient deaths only. Even more startling is the fact that this published article was based upon a report by the Institute of Medicine (IOM), which presented a much bleaker picture. If you look at the figures in the IOM report, which tracked both inpatient and outpatient deaths, you will find that the number of deaths caused by physician error jumps from 225,000 to around 284,000 per year.

Even if one is fortunate enough to survive such alarming errors, the subsequent health care burden is overwhelming. The *Journal of American Medicine* article provided the following glimpse into the after-effects of physician and medication error:

116 million extra doctor visits each year

77 million extra prescriptions per year

17 million hospital emergency room visits every year

8 million additional hospital admissions per year

3 million long-term admissions each year

199,000 additional deaths each and every year

$77 billion in extra costs—yes, every year

Each year, as many as twenty to thirty percent of Americans who seek medical care receive inappropriate care; an estimated 98,000 of these people die as a result of medical error associated with this inappropriate care. The shocking truth is that in a comparison of thirteen countries, the United States ranked next to dead last for sixteen available health indicators.

Certainly, it is not this book's intention to demean or bring into question the invaluable contributions that physicians and medical research have provided to our society. Their roles in treating what were previously incurable diseases have extended human life and, many times, enriched our longevity.

The issue, however, is that as a society we have become completely reliant on chemicals and medical procedures to cure all our ills without considering their potential aftermath. As demonstrated by the above statistics, this blindly unquestioning complacency is exacting a high toll in human suffering and loss of life. It is time to reclaim control of our health by learning more about the natural alternatives at our disposal.

Knowledge Is Power, But Only If You Apply It

Now that you know the potentially deadly hazards of prescription drugs and medical error, what is the next step? As you read on in this book, you will learn about the amazingly powerful role that natural nutrition can play in reclaiming your good health and then maintaining it.

Our bodies were created to heal themselves

naturally through the wonderful cornucopia of minerals, vitamins, and phytonutrients offered by our glorious planet. Everything we need to live—and live well—can be found in its plants, water, and minerals.

So why wait? Plug into the power of good nutrition and discover just how good you can feel, naturally.

CHAPTER TWO
Why Are We Fat?

Basic Causes of Obesity

To most people, obesity means being very overweight. In actuality, the term "overweight" indicates an excess amount of body weight including muscle, bone, fat, and water. Obesity, on the other hand, refers strictly to an excess amount of body fat. Athletes such as bodybuilders who have a lot of lean muscle tissue can be overweight, but would certainly never be considered obese. Obesity refers to being more than twenty percent over the ideal weight for your body structure, gender, and age.

You might be surprised to learn that at least eighty percent of adult Americans weigh more than they should, and half of these people are considered clinically obese.

In 1980, forty-six percent of American adults were overweight. By 2000, that figure had ballooned to sixty-four and a half percent, nearly a one percent annual increase in the number of overweight U.S. citizens. If this rate holds, by 2040, a horrifying one hundred percent of American adults will be overweight. Imagine! At the current rate of our national weight gain, in less than forty years every man, woman, and child in this country is projected to be overweight or obese.

Although some obesity is caused by underlying disorders, the main cause is probably lifestyle. Unfortunately, in the hectic, modern lifestyles common to our society, we tend to put taste and convenience before nutrition. Today, American society is all about bigger...bigger homes, bigger cars, and bigger meals. We eat much larger portions than our bodies really need while exercising much less than our bodies require.

Diets made up of high-calorie, high-sodium, and high-fat "fast foods" make it far too easy to quickly gain excess weight. Compounding this health problem is the fact that our sedentary lifestyles lack adequate exercise, making it incredibly hard to take that excess weight off. The result? An increasingly overweight nation.

You may remember the young man who became his own "human guinea pig" in an experiment to conclusively prove or disprove the theory that fast foods are harmfully unhealthy. He ate nothing but fast food for thirty consecutive days. Breakfast, lunch, dinner, and snacks all came from McDonald's. At the end of his thirty-day experiment, this young man's body was literally in a state of shambles. Although he was considered very healthy just a short thirty days earlier, he now suffered from extreme chronic fatigue and headaches, his blood sugar skyrocketed, his cholesterol levels and blood pressure became perilously high, and he gained twenty-five pounds of body fat—all in just thirty days.

New evidence does suggest that obesity may have more than one cause, though. Genetic, environmental, psychological, and other factors may all play a part in the obesity epidemic.

Obesity tends to run in families, which strongly suggests a genetic cause. And yet, families also tend to share diet and lifestyle habits that can certainly contribute to obesity. Separating these lifestyle habits from genetic factors is often quite difficult, but science does show that heredity is closely linked to obesity.

The good news, however, is that your gene pool does not necessarily condemn you to a lifetime of obesity. Environment also strongly influences a tendency toward obesity. This includes lifestyle behaviors such as the type and amount of foods you eat as well as your level of physical activity. The issue of environment can reinforce either learned poor eating behaviors or the decision to make healthier choices for yourself and your family.

Psychological factors can also influence eating habits. For example, many people eat in response to negative emotions such as boredom, sadness, or anger. Most overweight people have no more psychological problems than people of average weight, yet up to ten percent of mildly obese people who are trying to lose weight on their own or through structured weight-loss programs have a binge-eating disorder. This disorder is even more common in people who are severely obese. Those with the most severe binge-eating problems typically have symptoms of depression and low self-esteem and have more difficulty in losing weight and keeping it off than people without binge-eating problems.

Poor Eating Habits Don't Just Make You Fat

Twenty years ago, people weighing 300 pounds were a rarity. Now they are almost common. Childhood obesity, also once rare, has mushroomed to the point that fifteen percent of children between the ages of six and nineteen are considered overweight. And ten percent of our children who are between the ages of two and five are overweight. *At this rate, this may be the first generation of children who will die before their parents.*

The fact is that excess weight has been directly linked to a significantly increased risk of heart disease, stroke or other cardiovascular disease, diabetes, and several types of cancer, as well as sleep apnea, Alzheimer's disease, arthritis, infertility, gallstones, and asthma.

Heart disease and stroke are the leading causes of death and disability for both men and women in the United States. People who are chronically overweight are far more likely to have high blood pressure, a major risk factor for heart disease and stroke, than those who are not overweight. Also, excessively high levels of cholesterol and triglycerides are known causes of heart disease and are often linked to being overweight. Being overweight also contributes to angina, which is chest pain caused by decreased oxygen to the heart, as well as sudden death from heart disease or stroke—often without any signs or symptoms.

Type 2 diabetes is the most common type of diabetes in the United States, and its occurrence is growing at an incredibly alarming rate. Type 2 diabetes reduces your body's ability to control blood-sugar levels and is a major cause of early death, heart disease, kidney disease, stroke, and blindness. People who are overweight or obese are twice as likely to develop Type 2 diabetes as those who are not overweight.

Several types of cancer are now known to be associated with being overweight. In women, these include cancer of the uterus, gallbladder, cervix, ovary, breast, and colon. Overweight men are at great risk of developing cancer of the colon, rectum, and prostate.

Sleep apnea is a serious condition closely associated with being overweight. This condition can cause you to stop breathing for short periods while asleep and has also been directly linked to daytime sleepiness and fatigue. The real danger of sleep apnea is that it is also known to be a precursor to heart failure. The risk of suffering this potentially deadly condition increases with higher body weights.

Because Alzheimer's disease has been linked to obesity, the incidence of this memory-robbing neurological disease is on the rise. While genetic inheritance does play a role in Alzheimer's disease, factors associated with obesity such as diabetes and high cholesterol are known to significantly contribute to susceptibility. Many health professionals fear that the number of diagnosed Alzheimer's disease cases will likely triple in the next forty years as our nation becomes increasingly overweight.

Up to this point, ongoing improvements in medical care have dramatically reduced disability among older Americans and have even increased our longevity. But our continuing rate of unhealthy weight gain is creating a national health disaster that has the potential to undo many, if not all, of these advances in health care.

On the flip side of obesity, it is shocking to realize that doctors are beginning to see young girls suffering from osteoporosis and even arthritis. The reason is that, in their desperate desire to conform to our society's perceived image of beauty, these children are going on starvation diets. Instead of providing their growing bodies with the nutrition needed to develop healthy skeletal structures and musculature, they are drinking diet soft drinks and calling it a meal.

Excess Weight Also Impedes Proper Elimination

Excessive weight gain accompanied by a sedentary lifestyle can cause your metabolism to slow to a snail's pace. And while you continue to eat several large meals each day, fecal waste from all those meals is building up in your digestive system.

Think of it this way. If a person consumes one pound of food three times per day, but only goes to the bathroom once a day or once every two to three days, what do you suppose will happen? Chronic constipation. Constipation can result in up to five pounds of toxic fecal matter being stored in the intestinal system.

This build-up of toxic matter in your digestive tract not only results in additional weight gain, it sets the stage for a myriad of infections and even cancer. Additionally, excessive fecal matter build-up is known to actually coat the interior of your intestinal tract, making it practically impossible for good nutrients to be absorbed.

Any beneficial nutrients you consume end up being trapped within this fecal matter rather than helping to sustain the functions of your internal organs. You begin feeling listless and fatigued; your skin and hair take on a lifeless, generally unhealthy pallor; and you continue to gain weight, particularly in the belly region.

Why Food Cravings Get the Best of Us

What you must understand is that the body

craves what it needs, whether protein, fiber, vitamins, or minerals. The interesting thing is that the body remembers the foods that it has processed. So if your body craves a hot dog, for example, it is because it previously derived some form of protein from a hot dog. Your body does not care if that hot dog is junk food filled with fat and other harmful ingredients; it craves it as a recognized protein source.

You end up with overwhelming cravings for things filled with empty calories that you know are not good for you—and your waistline and overall body weight show it. Worse yet, your body *still* craves the nutrients it needs, so those cravings continue and even increase.

On the other hand, when you provide your body with fresh, wholesome food packed with the nutrients it needs, cravings subside, total caloric intake goes down, and weight loss becomes much easier.

Another known cause of food cravings is stress. The human body is designed to handle everything that comes at it, whether pleasure and relaxation or stress and anxiety. We each have hormones whose presence is increased or decreased, depending on the amount of stress present, by our bodies to handle everyday life. The problem with this is that it takes energy—energy that comes from caloric output. And when the body has been filled with nutrient-deficient calories, cravings immediately follow. As mentioned earlier, your body is always going to crave what it needs, which in this case is energy-producing nutrition.

So is there a solution? What can we, as a nation and as individuals, do to reverse these deadly cycles of poor nutrition and associated declining health? The answer is found in nature itself. Each and every one of us was created with the potential to be healthy and therefore have within us the capacity to enjoy a healthy, fulfilling life. The secret is to tap into the good health provided through nature's powerful vitamins, minerals, and phytonutrients.

Nature's nutritional bounty truly has a vital part to play in a modern society where our health is being constantly undermined by stress, pollution, pesticides, and too many fat-laden fast-food meals.

CHAPTER THREE
The Wellness Revolution

The Quest for a Healthier, Longer Life

As the leading edge of the baby-boomer generation approaches the age of retirement, their resounding attitude seems to be "we will not go quietly into the night." Indeed, these Americans whose revolutionary generation continuously defied the conventions of previous generations are now changing the face of retirement. Unwilling to spend days in a rocking chair with prescription bottles at hand, baby-boomers are actively seeking ways to live longer, healthier, more active lives. With the current predicted lifespan of between seventy-five to eighty-five years, baby-boomers are actively searching for ways to increase their quality of heath, endurance, and longevity—without the side effects of prescription drugs. They are searching for the proverbial "fountain of youth."

This ongoing quest for a longer, healthier life has given birth to another kind of revolution—the wellness revolution.

Generally speaking, baby-boomers simply don't plan to embrace the sedentary, elderly lifestyle of earlier generations. They are just not going to act old. The idea of whiling away their days with non-activity, much as their parents did, then lining up for the early-bird dinner special is not likely to have much of an appeal for the vast majority of baby-boomers. Indeed, more and more members of the largest age group in America (around 76 million strong) plan to become more active. They plan to travel...start a second career or business...learn to play a musical instrument...and become increasingly valuable members of society.

Their burning desire to look younger, feel better, and live longer has fueled research into the essential role of vitamins, minerals, and phytonutrients in regaining and maintaining vibrant good health. The results of this research are both startling and very elementary. Could it really be that nature has truly provided a "medicine chest" that heals, maintains glowing good health, and extends life?

Understanding That Chemicals May Not Be the Answer

At least five billion prescriptions will be filled this year in the United States alone. That figure averages out to around one and a half prescriptions every month for every man, woman and child in the United States. Annually, we spend approximately *two trillion dollars* for health care that primarily focuses on the treatment of disease rather than the promotion of good health and prevention of disease.

The sad truth is that, as we discussed in the previous chapter, the multitude of chemical drugs flowing into American homes is actually contributing to chronic illness, debilitation, and even premature death. These prescription drugs are all too often responsible for both fatal and non-fatal disorders. Many times, patients take handfuls of these drugs every day without really understanding the risks of potentially harmful interactions or disastrous side effects.

And with so many prescription drugs now available in a generic form, a shocking new danger has emerged. Most people are unaware that there is a twenty-five percent variance in generic prescription drugs, meaning that any generic prescription you have filled can either be twenty-five percent less potent or even twenty-five percent more potent than as stated on the label, depending on the manufacturer.

The reason this is such an important variable

is that each person's health affects the efficacy of a drug. What works on one person may have no effect on another, or its effectiveness can even vary from refill to refill for the same person.

Use of drugs prescribed by personal physicians to their patients is the third-leading cause of death in hospitals today, and drug-to-drug interactions are the eighth-leading cause of death. These horrifying statistics make it quite apparent that there is a very dark, dangerous underside to this proliferation of prescription "miracle" drugs.

The next time you notice a masterfully produced prescription drug commercial on television, pay close attention to the fine print and closing remarks. These hard-to-spot blurbs list possible side effects, and their disclosure is required by law. What you will discover are alarming side effects that many times are, quite honestly, worse than the conditions that the drugs are supposed to treat.

Believe it or not, there are people in the

world who do not rely upon medication to eliminate their symptoms, improve their health, reverse aging, or cure diseases. A growing army of people are realizing that "better living through chemicals" just isn't what it is cracked up to be. Instead, more and more people are turning to nature's "garden of health" to improve and sustain good health and vibrant energy, as well as to feel, think, and even look younger.

In a way, perhaps we as citizens of the planet Earth are rediscovering a natural fountain of youth that has always been right in front of us.

Returning to Nature for Improved Health and Increased Longevity

Everyone wants to live a long and healthy life. And although no one can guarantee how long we will live, a number of nutritional choices can markedly increase our chances of living into our eighties, nineties, or even longer.

For instance, did you know that six of the ten leading causes of death in the United States (coronary heart disease, stroke, cancer, diabetes, atherosclerosis, and liver disease) are associated with poor nutritional choices and overeating? This sobering information underscores the fact that good nutrition is one of the greatest weapons that we possess against disease.

Keeping unhealthy fats below thirty percent of the total calories you consume and your cholesterol intake below 200mg will significantly reduce your risk of heart disease.

Eating five servings per day of fruits and vegetables lowers your chances of getting cancer, and studies indicate that simply increasing the number of those servings to between nine and ten each day is as effective as prescription medication in lowering high blood pressure—without the dangerous side effects. This kind of superpowered natural nutrition can significantly reduce or even eliminate your risk of stroke.

Research scientists and even the American Medical Association all agree that nutritional supplements are absolutely essential to our health and wellbeing. Nowhere is this truer than when we consider our long-term health.

While our bodies are capable of healing themselves and keeping us healthy, they require a wide spectrum of nutrients to function properly and to remain healthy over a long life span. For complete nutrition, our bodies require vitamins, minerals, phytonutrients, trace minerals, enzymes, amino acids, essential fatty acids, and fiber. To further complicate the equation, these nutrients need to be in specific forms, and often in specific combinations, in order to provide optimum nutritional benefit.

It is extremely difficult for us to relate what we eat—or don't eat—today to what our health may be in five, ten, or even twenty years. You might even believe that aging and sickness are a natural part of life. However, the truth is that with the right nutritional choices—including anti-aging vitamins, minerals, and antioxidants—it is more than possible to restore and maintain good health while also slowing or even reversing the aging process.

If you are ready to feel better than you have in years, enjoy the kind of energy you had as a child and look years younger, then you definitely don't want to miss a single word of the next chapter: Nature's Medicine Chest!

CHAPTER FOUR
Nature's Medicine Chest

Benefits of Basic Good Nutrition

Your body is a temple, and what you put in it can quite literally determine how well that temple looks and functions and even plays a very large part in how long it lasts.

For example, with all that we now know about tobacco, why do people still smoke? The answer is surprisingly simple. Marketing makes smoking look cool, and it is very, very habit-forming. But consider this—poor nutritional choices are known to cause just as much incidence of cancer, disability, chronic disease, and even death as cigarettes do. As a matter of fact, the typical American diet of today is often cited as our number one public health threat.

We've discussed the disastrous effects of a diet filled with our beloved fast food. It has become widespread public knowledge that junk food is making us overweight and sick, and yet we continue our love affair with it. Why? Interestingly, most likely for the same reasons people continue to puff away on cigarettes—the marketing is overwhelmingly enticing with entertaining, delicious-looking advertising, and it is very, very habit-forming.

Proper nutrition significantly reduces your risk of a variety of health problems, including heart disease and cancer. To keep your body functioning at its very best with optimum energy, good health, and longevity, a diet high in fruits and vegetables is strongly recommended. You see, most fruits and vegetables have no cholesterol, fat, or sodium. While they are naturally occurring, these three compounds have a profoundly negative effect on your good health.

Fruits and vegetables are also rich in the vitamins and minerals that your body requires to function properly. As a matter of fact, practically every essential vitamin and mineral that you need to stay healthy can be found in nature's cornucopia of fruits and vegetables.

For example, vitamins A, C, and E can assist with the prevention of coronary artery disease by keeping plaque build-up from occurring on artery walls. Vitamin B-1 is needed for digestion and proper nervous system function. Vitamin B-2 is needed for normal cell growth. Vitamin B-3 helps detoxify your body. Folic acid assists with production of red blood cells. Vitamin D assists with the absorption of calcium. Vitamin K helps your blood clot.

Minerals and trace elements are two other nutrients that your body requires, as both are used in a number of different body processes. Minerals like chlorine help create your digestive juices, and phosphorus helps build strong bones.

Now let's talk a bit about antioxidants.

A great number of our health adversities can be directly traced to the distortion or corruption of oxygen. That's right; the very thing that gives life can also help take it away. Oxidants, toxic forms of oxygen that occur in our bodies at a cellular level, can cause normal cells to mutate into cancerous ones, clog arteries, cause joints and eyesight to deteriorate, and even cause the nervous system to seriously malfunction. In fact, scientists have linked these destructive oxygen reactions to more than sixty chronic diseases as well as to premature aging. Renegade oxidant molecules are also sometimes called "free radicals." Oxidant free radicals can attack DNA, the genetic material of cells, causing them to mutate into pre-cancerous cells. And science has discovered that these free radicals produce more free radicals that produce even more free radicals, all intent on destroying the healthy cells in their paths.

So where do these free radical molecules come from and how do they form? The major culprits are environmental pollution, smoking, drugs, and poor nutritional choices. The good news is that you can outwit dangerous free radicals by mounting an antioxidant defense.

By incorporating the right nutrition, particularly fruits and vegetables, into your daily diet, you can supply your cells with antioxidant food compounds that strike down, intercept, and even destroy rampaging oxidant molecules. Antioxidants can even repair some of the damage caused by these rogue free radicals.

Simple guidelines for a well-balanced, nutritional diet include at least two and a half cups of vegetables and two cups of fruit each day. When making your daily food selections, be sure to choose a good variety of these antioxidant-rich treasures. You should also eat at least three ounces of whole grain products each day. Your total fat intake should only be between ten to thirty percent of your daily calories. And remember that most of the fats you consume should be in the form of unsaturated fats, as saturated fats can do much to damage your health. Less than ten percent of your calories should come from saturated fats, and always try to avoid trans-fatty acid.

Fiber-rich fruits, vegetables, and whole grains should be a regular part of your diet, as should potassium-rich foods.

Nutrients That Can Prevent and Even Cure Common Illnesses

According to the World Health Organization, as much as eighty percent of the world's population relies on medicines made from natural ingredients. Indeed, nature's medicine chest offers a wealth of health-giving nutrients free from the dangers of harmful side effects so often associated with synthetically produced prescription drugs.

Degenerative Diseases

Degenerative diseases including cancer, heart disease, arthritis, and diabetes have overrun Western society and threaten to become a global epidemic. While degenerative diseases are usually associated with old age, old age is not the real cause. The real culprit is the lack of proper nutrition and the presence of undesirable substances, such as high-fat, high-sodium preservatives and chemicals in our modern food. In fact, most of today's degenerative diseases are the direct result of poor nutritional choices.

Arthritis

Chronic pain, inflammation, joint damage, and immobility are all associated with arthritis in its various crippling forms. However, a number of nutrients are known to pack a powerful punch against this cruelly debilitating disease.

Ginger has been found to be incredibly beneficial in the treatment of arthritis. It is, in fact, considered by many to be superior to widely prescribed anti-arthritis drugs known as NSAIDs (non-steroidal anti-inflammatory drugs), and even provides effective pain relief. But ginger is not the only arthritis-fighting spice. Turmeric and cloves are known to combat inflammation naturally as they improve morning stiffness and swollen joints. And pomegranates help to ease arthritis while also lowering blood pressure, preventing hardening of the arteries, and guarding against osteoporosis.

Another powerful nutrient that has enjoyed amazing success in relieving, reversing, and preventing crippling arthritis and other debilitating joint disorders is Omega-3 fatty acid. It is interesting to note that it takes more Omega-3 fatty acid to subdue arthritis than to prevent it. You may never be plagued with arthritis in the first place if you consistently make Omega-3 fatty acid a part of your daily diet.

Also appearing to be of great benefit are several other nutrients. For example, in a number of tests, glucosamine was found to be as effective as or more effective than ibuprofen for relief of arthritis symptoms. Chondroitin sulfate is a cartilage-building natural compound whose properties complement the benefits of glucosamine. Methylsulfonylmethane (MSM) is a naturally powerful sulfur compound that appears to inhibit pain impulses along nerve fibers, acting as an analgesic and anti-inflammatory. Niacinamide is a form of vitamin B3 that has been shown to be particularly effective in addressing knee pain associated with arthritis.

Cancer

Diet is now considered a major weapon in the fight against cancer, with the National Cancer Institute reporting that at least one-third, and more likely over one-half, of all cancers are linked to diet. For example, low levels of vitamin A and carotene increase the likelihood of cancer, particularly lung cancer. And low levels of vitamin C greatly increase the likelihood of stomach and gastro-intestinal cancer.

The one constant that researchers and doctors agree upon is that the more fruits and vegetables one consumes, the less likely that person is to get cancer—including colon, stomach, breast, ovary, pancreatic, bladder, and even lung cancer. Even more striking is the fact that those who consistently eat large amounts of fruits and vegetables have about half the risk of cancer as those who eat very few fruits and vegetables.

Some of the top cancer-fighting nutrients that definitely need to be a part of your daily nutrition are garlic, cabbage, soybeans, ginger, carrots, celery, onions, tea (preferably green, but black and oolong have anti-cancer effects as well), turmeric, grapefruit and other citrus fruits, tomatoes, broccoli, cauliflower, oregano, cucumber, potatoes, thyme, red grapes, raspberries, barley, and berries. Set a goal to include at least five, but preferably nine, servings of these cancer-fighting nutrients in your diet every day.

Also, don't skimp on calcium, magnesium, vitamin D, and vitamin C, as these nutrients possess incredibly powerful cancer-inhibiting properties.

Heart Disease

Here is some monumental news for anyone who is concerned about heart disease, including those who have already suffered a heart attack. Changing your nutritional choices right now can help prevent future cardiac catastrophe and even halt or reverse arterial damage while helping restore your arteries to good health.

Increasing the amount of fruits and vegetables in your daily diet can slash your chances of heart attack and stroke, even if you have already suffered one or the other. A large body of research supports the fact that foods rich in beta-carotene and other antioxidants can significantly reduce your risk of heart attack, and the incidence of stroke can be reduced by up to an amazing seventy percent.

So to keep the cardiologist away, here is some sound nutritional advice. A good heart-healthy diet needs to be low in salt and saturated fat, yet high in cardio-protective foods and nutrients including fiber, flaxseed, folate, magnesium, Omega-3 fatty acids, soy, and antioxidants such as lycopene, flavonoids, and vitamins C and E. Also, use extra-virgin olive oil or canola oil rather than corn oil. Go heavy on fruits and vegetables to keep your blood supply packed with plenty of the antioxidants and anticoagulants that protect your arteries from clogging.

Some of the most heart-friendly fruits and vegetables are broccoli, blueberries, pomegranates, carrots, barley, oats, apples, tomatoes, oranges, garlic, onions, strawberries, raspberries, grapefruit, spinach, asparagus, soybeans, Brussels sprouts, and beets.

Botanicals can also be powerful weapons in your fight against heart disease. Hawthorn is a botanical frequently prescribed as a heart remedy in Europe. A potent antioxidant, it appears to work by opening up blood vessels that feed the heart, thus increasing its energy supply and enhancing its pumping power. Another fabulously heart-healthy botanical is grape seed extract, which increases blood circulation and helps strengthen blood vessels.

High Cholesterol

High cholesterol has become a major health issue and is one of the leading contributors to heart disease. Rather than risk the dangerous side effects of statin drugs that reduce *all* cholesterol—both the bad LDL as well as the good HDL—there are several nutrients that have shown amazing abilities to reduce and even reverse existing artery-clogging cholesterol buildup. At the forefront of these marvelous nutrients is the humble garlic. If you are concerned about unhealthy cholesterol levels, garlic should definitely be a part of your daily diet. A number of published research studies show that garlic can and does reduce harmful LDL cholesterol by as much as fifteen percent. Equally exciting is the discovery that garlic dramatically raises the liver's production of beneficial HDL by twenty-three percent. [4] [5]

Other tasty nutrients that pack a cholesterol-reducing punch are onions, olive oil, almonds and walnuts, strawberries, avocados, apples, carrots, legumes such as beans and chickpeas, broccoli, oranges, apricots, grapefruit, and mangos. Each of these fruits and vegetables are rich in fabulous antioxidants that help keep your LDL cholesterol from becoming oxidized and toxic. Co-enzyme Q10 and Omega-3 fatty acids are also very powerful artery-protecting antioxidants.

Diabetes

By 2050, more than 48 million Americans will likely have some form of diabetes, which has already become the fifth leading cause of death in the United States. Diabetes greatly increases your risk of heart disease and kidney failure, as well as damage to your circulatory system and vision. The good news, though, is that diabetics who incorporate good nutritional choices as well as high-quality nutritional supplements into their daily diet typically report better health than those who do not.

So what nutrients are on the leading edge of reducing the effects of and even preventing diabetes?

Broccoli is a super source of chromium, a trace mineral that seems to work wonders on blood sugar. Barley is also rich in chromium, as are nuts, oysters, whole grains, and rhubarb. And don't forget to spice up your diet with cinnamon, cloves, and turmeric. These three kitchen favorites actually have drug-like properties that help stimulate insulin activity, helping your body to process sugar more efficiently. Interestingly, turmeric has demonstrated the ability to *triple* insulin activity. High-carbohydrate, high-fiber legumes are also very effective in keeping diabetes under control and even preventing it. High-fiber diets often work so well that many diabetics have been able to decrease or even eliminate their need for supplemental insulin and other anti-diabetic medications.

Osteoporosis

Osteoporosis is a silent epidemic that has already stricken over forty-four million Americans. In fact, fifty-five percent of those over the age of fifty have osteoporosis.

What exactly is osteoporosis, and why is it so dangerous? Osteoporosis is a disease without a known cure that ravages the body's bone structure. It is characterized by low bone mass and the progressive deterioration of bone tissue, particularly in the spine, hips, and wrists. The result is increasingly fragile bones that are easily fractured.

In advanced cases of osteoporosis, something as harmless as a sneeze can cause a vertebra to fracture. A fall can easily result in debilitating hip or spine fractures. And while hip fractures are most commonly associated with osteoporosis, any bone can be affected.

According to the National Osteoporosis Foundation, this silent disease was responsible for more than two million fractures in 2005. This figure is expected to skyrocket to over three million by 2025. Particularly alarming is the fact that approximately twenty-four percent of those persons who suffer an osteoporosis-associated hip fracture after the age of fifty die within a year following such an injury.

Diet plays an important part in our susceptibility to osteoporosis. Low calcium and vitamin D intake combined with a diet high in caffeine, sodium, and protein are sure to put you at high risk for osteoporosis. Smoking and prescription medications such as steroids are also known to significantly increase your risk.

To keep osteoporosis from affecting your quality of life and potentially shortening your life, be sure to include foods naturally high in calcium such as broccoli, oranges, cabbage, just about any kind of bean, almonds, and low-fat milk. Most health experts recommend that you incorporate 1,200mg of calcium as well as 800mg of vitamin D3 into your daily diet in order to keep your bones and teeth healthy.

Another important factor in avoiding the ravages of osteoporosis is to get up and get moving! Incorporate daily walks or some other kind of weight-bearing exercise into your regular routine.

Alzheimer's Disease

In the next forty years, the number of people suffering the memory-robbing ravages of Alzheimer's disease is expected to triple. And because obesity has been linked to Alzheimer's, that figure may grow even higher. Over-medication and vitamin deficiencies also significantly contribute to impaired memory. However, making good nutritional choices right now can help protect the health of your brain and keep your mind sharp.

Your brain function can definitely be boosted by feeding your mind the nutrients it craves. For example, high-fiber foods such as fruits, vegetables, nuts, and whole grains appear to protect against Alzheimer's. Also, several studies indicate that green tea helps prevent inflammation and brain cell damage. Essential fatty acids like Omega-3 help prevent cognitive decline as we age, but you should avoid Omega-6 fats found in highly processed corn oil as they have been linked to cognitive decline.

Ginkgo, ginger, and turmeric are three botanicals that are "must-haves" in your brain-healthy diet. Ginkgo, rich in flavonoids, increases blood flow to the brain and enhances the ability to focus while also reducing inflammation and free radical damage to brain cells. Adding anti-inflammatory ginger appears to provide even more protection against age-related mental decline. Turmeric contains antioxidant and anti-inflammatory properties that inhibit cognition-disruptive plaque buildup and actually breaks up existing plaque.

Adequate supplies of the nutrients alpha

lipoic acid; vitamins A, C, and E; acetyl-L-carnitine; and phosphatidylserine are also vital in protecting yourself from dementia, a variety of cognitive dysfunctions, and Alzheimer's disease.

Depression, Anxiety, and Other Mood Disorders

Each year, depression, anxiety, and other mood disorders afflict over thirty percent of the world's population. While the typical treatment involves prescription drugs, this approach merely masks the symptoms rather than addressing the root cause. So to alleviate depression safely and permanently, it is crucial to correct any chemical imbalance within the body. Research shows us that it is entirely possible to correct this imbalance by revising nutrient intake. Amazingly, a deficiency of any one nutrient can alter brain function and lead to depression, anxiety, and other mental disorders. It is then no surprise that one of the most common threads found among people who suffer from depression and other mental disorders is their poor nutritional habits.

Deficiencies of specific nutrients are quite common in depressed individuals. The most common deficiencies are folic acid (also known as vitamin B-9), vitamins B-12 and B-6, and Omega 3 essential fatty acids. Increasing the levels of these nutrients offers a natural and remarkably effective way to positively influence depression, anxiety, and other mood disorders.

Additionally, complex carbohydrates found in whole grains as well as fresh fruits and vegetables have been shown to help sustain a long-lasting flow of the dietary amino acid tryptophan—which, in turn, creates the mood-lifting hormone serotonin—to the blood and brain.

Treating depression through this type of proper nutrition is one of the most effective and safe ways to put brain chemistry back in balance and break free from the chains of depression.

Common Cold

The first thing that comes to mind when treating the common cold is that taking vitamin C will help, and this instinct is correct. Two-time Nobel Prize winner and nutritional visionary Linus Pauling first discovered the connection between vitamin C and the common cold, and today most naturopaths agree that this is an excellent first step in warding off a cold. Zinc is also recommended for those just beginning to come down with a cold. It is not only an important regulator of immunity, but is also an excellent mineral to take in the event of viral illness, which is exactly what the common cold is. So load up on citrus fruits and keep your body hydrated with plenty of pure, filtered water.

Also, foods rich in beta-carotene such as sweet potatoes, dark and leafy greens, broccoli, and squash are particularly helpful in soothing cold-inflamed mucus membranes. And the herb echinacea is valued for its wonderful immune-enhancing properties that can help you prevent or even recover from a cold.

As you can see, nature has quite literally provided her human occupants with everything needed to become and stay healthy. The amazing vitamins, minerals, and phytonutrients found in her bountiful "medicine chest" offer up incredible good health, clarity of mind, and increased longevity. Want to learn more about the fabulous benefits of nature's vitamins, minerals, and phytonutrients? Then read on!

CHAPTER FIVE
The ABCs of Nutritional Vitamins and Minerals

Vitamins and minerals are now universally recognized as playing a huge role in the health and vitality of every organ in the body, from your skin and bones to your nervous and immune systems to even your brain. Studies have shown that being well nourished with vitamins and minerals can dramatically lower harmful cholesterol levels, help wounds heal faster, help bulletproof the body against debilitating and even deadly diseases, raise men's sperm count, and help fight off those nasty colds as well as the flu, asthma, cataracts, and even gum disease.

The Astonishing Power of Vitamins

Most people don't realize just how crucial vitamins are to their health. Unlike macronutrients such as dietary fats, carbohydrates, and proteins, vitamins regulate metabolic reactions. In other words, you can consume just the right amounts of fats, carbohydrates, and proteins and even exercise like a maniac, but unless your body also has a good supply of vitamins to regulate how these macronutrients are used, very little benefit will be gained from them. In fact, the absence of just a single vitamin can block one or more metabolic reactions, eventually disrupting your entire metabolic balance at a cellular level.

Here is a quick overview of the incredible health benefits provided by specific vitamins.

Vitamin A: Sometimes referred to as beta-carotene, vitamin A is fat-soluble vitamin that serves several major functions in your body. It helps cells reproduce normally, is required for normal fetal growth and development, and is needed for normal reproductive function. Vitamin A is also required for vision as it maintains healthy cells in various structures of the eye and is essential for the transfer of light into nerve signals in the retina. It helps regulate your immune system, plays a major role in bone growth, and helps maintain the surface linings of the respiratory, urinary, and intestinal tracts. When these linings break down, bacteria and viruses can enter the body and cause infection. The earliest sign of vitamin A deficiency is poor night vision, but other symptoms can include dry skin, increased risk of infections, and metaplasia, which is a dangerous pre-cancerous condition.

Vitamin B-1: Also known as thiamine, vitamin B-1 is necessary for practically every cellular reaction in the body. It is vital for normal functioning of the nervous system, heart, muscles, and metabolism. Vitamin B-1 works with other B vitamins to release the energy from food you consume and also helps maintain the health of your mucus membranes. Additionally, it supports normal growth and development and reduces depression, fatigue, and even motion sickness. Symptoms of vitamin B-1 deficiency include fatigue, depression, decreased mental functioning, muscle cramps, nausea, heart enlargement, and eventually beriberi.

Vitamin B-2: Otherwise known as riboflavin, vitamin B-2 is essential to energy generation, nerve development, blood-cell development, and the regulation of certain hormones. It also plays an important role in normal growth and development as well as keeping your brain and nervous system healthy. Together with vitamins A and B-1, vitamin B-2 supports the health of your mucus membranes, skin, and even your hair. Symptoms of a vitamin B-2 deficiency can include red, swollen, or cracked mouth and tongue tissue; fatigue; depression; and anemia. The formation of cataracts may be a result of this vitamin deficiency.

Vitamin B-3: Also known as cholecalciferol, vitamin B-3 acts like other B vitamins to create enzymes that are essential to metabolic cell activity. It synthesizes hormones, repairs genetic material, and maintains normal functioning of the nervous system. Vitamin B-3 is also known to decrease harmful cholesterol and triglyceride levels as it helps keep your blood vessels dilated to ensure healthy blood flow. This fabulous vitamin is essential for the repair of genetic material; helps ward off heart attacks, depression, and migraine headaches; and can even help improve digestion and increase the absorption of calcium. Vitamin B-3 deficiency can produce symptoms such as dermatitis on the hands and face, weakness, loss of appetite, sore mouth, diarrhea, anxiety, depression, osteoporosis, and even dementia.

Vitamin B-5: Also called pantothenic acid, vitamin B-5 is a co-enzyme involved in energy metabolism of carbohydrates, protein, and fat. Like vitamin B-2, vitamin B-5 is crucial to normal growth and development. It also helps relieve stress, reduces fatigue, and even helps promote wound healing. Symptoms of vitamin B-5 deficiency include excessive fatigue, sleep disturbances, loss of appetite, nausea, or dermatitis.

Vitamin B-6: Pyridoxine, also known as vitamin B-6, helps carry out metabolic processes that affect your body's utilization of protein, carbohydrates, and fat. It is also vital to the maintenance of a healthy nervous system and produces the mood-regulating hormone serotonin. Vitamin B-6 promotes cardiovascular health and helps reduce painful inflammation associated with arthritis, carpal tunnel syndrome and other musculoskeletal conditions, and has even been linked to the reduction of PMS and asthma symptoms. It is key in the formation of hemoglobin in red blood cells and antibodies that help fight infection and anemia. Symptoms of vitamin B-6 deficiency include weakness, mental confusion, irritability, nervousness, inability to sleep, hyperactivity, anemia, skin lesions, tongue discoloration, and kidney stones.

Vitamin B-9: More commonly known as folic acid, vitamin B-9 is crucial for proper cell replication and growth. Folic acid forms building blocks of DNA, the body's genetic information, and building blocks of RNA, which are needed for protein synthesis in all cells. Rapidly growing tissues such as those of a fetus and rapidly regenerating cells like red blood cells and immune cells have a high need for folic acid. Vitamin B-9 reduces the risk of spina bifida during pregnancy and works with vitamin B-12 to help keep the circulation healthy. Another exciting discovery about folic acid is that it may help fight against several types of cancer and cardiovascular disease. Symptoms of folic acid deficiency include anemia, mood disorders, and gastrointestinal disorders. Neural tube defects may occur when a vitamin B-9 deficiency occurs during pregnancy.

Vitamin B-12: Also known as cyanocobalamin, vitamin B-12 is needed for normal nerve cell activity, DNA replication, and production of the mood-affecting hormone SAMe (S-adenosyl-L-methionine). Vitamin B-12 acts with folic acid and vitamin B-6 to reduce the risk of heart disease, stroke, osteoporosis, and Alzheimer's disease. And, of course, vitamin B-12 is famous for its ability to quickly increase energy and memory. Symptoms of a vitamin B-12 deficiency include nausea, loss of appetite, sore mouth, diarrhea, loss of sensation in hands and feet, confusion, memory loss, and depression. Harmful anemia can also be a result of this deficiency.

Vitamin C: One of the most crucial vitamins in your body, vitamin C plays a large role in hundreds of the body's functions. This powerful antioxidant helps to protect against free radicals; fights infection; boosts iron absorption; and helps maintain healthy skin, blood vessels, bones, and gums. It is also essential for the manufacture of collagen, which is vital for tissue repair. Vitamin C even helps heal wounds, burns, and broken tissues. It contributes to hemoglobin and production of red blood cells in bone marrow and is effective against urinary tract infections and anemia. Even more exciting is the fact that vitamin C promotes production of interferon, a compound that is known to fight cancer. Symptoms of vitamin C deficiency include prolonged healing of wounds, frequent infections, prolonged colds, muscle weakness, loss of teeth, bleeding gums, swollen or painful joints, nosebleeds, bruising, anemia, and depression.

Vitamin D: Sometimes called the sunshine vitamin, vitamin D is needed for normal body growth and development. In particular, vitamin D helps your body absorb calcium and phosphorus to create bone. Vitamin D plays a role in maintaining a healthy immune system and blood cell formation and also helps cells "differentiate"—a process that may reduce the risk of cancer. It is needed to produce and maintain adequate blood levels of insulin. Deficiency symptoms include bone pain and tenderness and muscle weakness. In children, rickets may occur, in which bones lose calcium and become soft and curved. Without proper daily intake of vitamin D, there is an increased risk of osteoporosis, arthritis, and cancer.

Vitamin E: Also known as alpha tocopherol, vitamin E is an antioxidant that protects cell membranes and other fat-soluble parts of the body, such as LDL cholesterol (the "bad" cholesterol), from damage. Only when LDL is damaged does cholesterol appear to lead to heart disease, and vitamin E is an important antioxidant protector of LDL. In addition to its antioxidant functions, vitamin E is known to have a positive effect on inflammation, blood cell regulation, connective tissue growth, and genetic control of cell division. It also plays a role in the body's ability to process glucose. Symptoms of vitamin E deficiency include lethargy, loss of balance, and anemia. There may even be an increased risk of heart disease, cancer, and premature aging with marginal deficiencies of this vitamin.

Vitamin H: Also referred to as biotin, vitamin H is a water-soluble B vitamin that assists in the metabolism of protein, fats, and carbohydrates. It is also important in the transfer of carbon dioxide. Biotin even helps maintain a steady blood sugar level. Symptoms of a vitamin H deficiency, although rare, may include hair loss, dermatitis, anemia, muscle pain, loss of appetite, lethargy, depression, hallucinations, and lowered immunity.

Vitamin K: Phytonadione, more commonly known as vitamin K, promotes normal blood clotting. It is also essential for proper kidney function and plays an important role in normal growth and development. Symptoms of vitamin K deficiency include prolonged clotting time, easy bleeding, and bruising.

Those Magnificent Minerals

All of our bodily processes are dependent on the action of minerals, with the proper efficiency of each mineral being enhanced by balanced amounts of other minerals as well as vitamins. For example, the mineral zinc is required for your body to convert vitamin A into its active form. And without vitamin A in its active form, a variety of problems quickly manifest, such as vision deterioration. When our bodies cannot continuously produce healthy cells due to the lack of certain minerals, the result can be premature aging, the development of chronic and debilitating diseases and, in some cases, even instances of early death.

Calcium: No other mineral is capable of performing as many biological functions as calcium. This amazing mineral provides the electrical energy that keeps your heart beating as well as your muscles moving. And while calcium is certainly famous as a vital bone protector, it plays other important roles as well, helping your nerve cells to communicate and your blood to clot normally. Calcium also helps lower blood pressure, and even helps prevent colon cancer and premenstrual syndrome. Another important biological job for calcium is DNA replication, which is crucial for maintaining a youthful and healthy body. As important as all these and hundreds of other biological functions of calcium are to human health, none is more important than the job of pH control. One of the most effective and easily absorbed forms of calcium is *coral calcium,* which is discussed at more length in a later chapter.

Chromium: Helps insulin work more efficiently, making it an especially important nutrient for people who have Type 2 diabetes or are at risk for it. Insulin usually helps lower blood sugar levels, but if you have Type 2 diabetes, your insulin is considerably less effective. In fact, some cases of Type 2 diabetes are triggered by a chromium deficiency. Interestingly, chromium's effect on insulin may also help you lose weight.

Iodine: Essential in the production of thyroid hormones, which regulate your body's metabolic rate. It also plays a key role in vital bodily functions such as body temperature, growth, and development; the manufacture of healthy blood cells; and even nerve and muscle function.

Iron: The main function of iron is found in hemoglobin, which is the part of red blood cells that carry oxygen from the lungs to all the cells in your body. If the body runs short of iron, iron-deficiency anemia develops with symptoms including tiredness, irritability, and reduced resistance to infection. Women in particular need to be sure to include enough iron in their daily diet.

Magnesium: Essential for hundreds of chemical reactions that occur in the body every second of every day. Its health-promoting benefits include the ability to prevent heart disease as well as treat chronic conditions such as fibromyalgia and diabetes. Magnesium works with calcium to maintain healthy bones, helps release energy from food and absorb its nutrients, and even plays a role in regulating mood as well as nerve and muscle function.

Phosphorous: Often considered a twin nutrient to calcium due to its powerful contribution to bone health. It is an essential mineral so abundant in the body that the average person normally retains about a pound and a half of it. Phosphorous is involved, either directly or indirectly, in nearly every biological or cellular function in the body. Working together with calcium, phosphorous builds and hardens bones and teeth. It is also required to help maintain the blood's acid balance, or pH. It strengthens cell walls and supports the transport of nutrients and various hormones throughout the body.

Potassium: With the exception of calcium and phosphorus, no other mineral is as abundant in the human body as potassium, which is essential to the regulation of blood pressure and muscle contraction and helps keep nerves, kidneys, and a host of other body processes functioning properly. A healthy intake of potassium is valuable for general health and can even help to maintain normal blood pressure. In fact, according to various studies, it offers significant protection against heart disease and stroke.

Selenium: One of our most potent allies in the fight against cancer. This powerful antioxidant appears to regenerate vitamins E and C, enabling them to continue fighting free radicals.

The results of one double-blind study which lasted four and a half years indicate that participants who took 200mcg of selenium per day reduced their risk of cancer by a full thirty-two percent, and the risk of death from cancer by a stunning fifty percent.[6]

Trace minerals: Part of DNA, our genetic material. A number of trace minerals—including boron, fluoride, manganese, molybdenum, silicon, and vanadium—aid in growth and development. Other trace minerals promote the formation of strong bones and connective tissues and help to prevent osteoporosis. This strengthening property also protects against strains and sprains. In addition, a number of trace minerals show amazing potential to guard against heart disease and control seizures, among other beneficial actions.

Zinc: An essential trace mineral. Every cell in your body needs this nutrient and hundreds of body processes rely upon it, from the immune system and the enzymes that produce DNA to the senses of taste and smell. It helps keep the skin healthy, aids wound healing, and is particularly important during pregnancy and infant development. A zinc deficiency in adulthood has been linked to increased risk of infection, skin and hair problems, and a low sperm count.

Fruits and Vegetables Burst with Vitamins and Minerals—Naturally

So now that you know how incredibly vital vitamins and minerals are to your health, how do you find them? And will they taste dreadful? Most of us simply will not gnaw on a rock for the sake of minerals, so how do you give your body what it requires for optimum health?

The answer lies in beautifully colorful, mouth-wateringly tasty fruits and vegetables. You see, fruits and vegetables are naturally bursting with life-giving vitamins and minerals called phytonutrients. Here's a quick look at some of the nutritional superstars of the plant kingdom.

Beta-carotene and related compounds called carotenoids are converted by the body to vitamin A. Carotenoids (from the word "carrot") are found in high concentrations in carrots, other orange and yellow vegetables, and fruits such as winter squash and cantaloupes. Dark, green, leafy vegetables—such as spinach, kale, broccoli, and other members of the cabbage family—also contain high concentrations of carotenoids.

Dark green vegetables as well as oranges, beets, and raspberries are excellent sources of folic acid, vitamins E and K, and minerals such as calcium, magnesium, manganese, iron, and potassium. Many fruits are also good sources of minerals such as chromium (grapes), iron (cherries), manganese (pineapple), and potassium (apricots, bananas, oranges, peaches, and prunes).

Exotic fruits such as mangosteen, noni, mangos, papaya, star fruit and goji berries are loaded with vitamins such as E, C, B-1, and B-6.

Another exotic fruit that has been receiving increased attention for its nutritional benefits is gac fruit. Now, you have likely never heard of this odd-sounding fruit, but it has been a market favorite in Asia for many years. Gac fruit is particularly high in lycopene, which is an effective cancer-fighting nutrient that we usually only think of when it comes to tomatoes. However, gac fruit contains up to seventy times the amount of lycopene found in tomatoes.[7] This odd little fruit is also packed with beta-carotene.

Now let's talk about another little known exotic fruit called cili. It is believed that the cili fruit has more vitamin C than any other fruit typically associated with this vitamin. Just how much vitamin C are we talking about? Perhaps as much as sixty times more than oranges!

All of these fabulous exotic fruits also provide a bonanza of the beneficial minerals that your body requires.

Citrus fruits are good sources of vitamin C, as is the family of plants including tomatoes, red and green peppers, potatoes, and eggplant. Other good sources of vitamin C include papayas, strawberries, kiwis, cantaloupe, and the cabbage family, including broccoli, cauliflower, and Brussels sprouts.

Nuts are a fabulous source of vitamin E, as are whole-grain wheat, soybeans, and lima beans. And the richest vegetable sources of calcium include collard greens, figs, kale, broccoli, okra, horseradish, soybeans, celery, cabbage, chickpeas, red kidney beans, and pinto beans.

Looking for foods to pump up your potassium? Delicious cantaloupe, avocados, peaches, prunes, tomatoes, soybeans, apricots, Swiss chard, oranges, pumpkin, sweet potatoes, bananas, acorn squash, almonds, spinach, and peanuts are all rich in this fabulous phytonutrient.

Brazil nuts, sunflower seeds, whole-grain wheat, and garlic are famous for their selenium content, while red peppers, green peppers, cantaloupe, papaya, strawberries, Brussels sprouts, grapefruit, kiwi fruit, oranges, tomatoes, broccoli, cauliflower, green peas, and kale are incredibly rich in zinc.

Don't Forget The Benefits Of Sea Veggies!

Most people just don't think about the ocean when talking about vegetables, yet the deep blue sea offers up a vast source of nutrition. Sea vegetables are virtually fat-free and low in calories; surprisingly, they are also some of the richest sources of minerals in the plant kingdom. Sea vegetables contain high amounts of calcium and phosphorous, and are extremely high in magnesium, iron, iodine, and sodium. They also contain vitamins A, B-1, C, and E, as well as protein and carbohydrates.

Together, these nutrients make sea vegetables a potent and valuable weapon against a myriad of nutritional deficiencies directly linked to cancer, heart disease, diabetes, arthritis, and scores of other frighteningly debilitating health issues.

But sea vegetables are not the only nutritional treasures the ocean has to offer. In the next chapter, you will discover the amazing secret to increased longevity and incredible good health hidden in the depths of Okinawa's sparkling blue seas.

CHAPTER SIX
The Sea's Surprising Treasure Trove of Calcium

As we discussed earlier, one of the most important of elements in the human body is calcium. It is one of the most abundant minerals in the human body, and accounts for approximately one and a half percent of our total body weight. Bones and teeth comprise ninety-nine percent of the calcium in our bodies, with the remaining one percent distributed in other areas.

However, it is also a mineral that is alarmingly lacking in the typical Western diet. Sadly, this calcium deficiency can have devastating consequences.

In fact, up to 150 diseases have been directly linked to calcium deficiency. A lack of it in the blood stream can cause seizures, heart irregularities, muscle cramps, diarrhea or constipation, and even major disruptions in the brain's functions—causing memory loss, unclear thinking, and loss of consciousness.

In recent years, American consumers have been bombarded with public health messages encouraging the consumption of calcium-rich foods. The purpose of these messages is to help stem the rapidly increasing incidence of osteoporosis, a disease characterized by brittle and porous bones that afflicts more than forty-four million individuals in the United States. As mentioned in a previous chapter, a calcium-deficient diet has been identified as one of the primary causative factors of this devastating disease.

Calcium, sometimes called the "king of minerals" protects our bodies in a myriad of ways, including bulletproofing our skeletal structures against osteoporosis and other debilitating bone and joint diseases.

As essential as this mineral is to our health, calcium in its inland form is one of the most difficult minerals for our bodies to absorb.

The Secret of Okinawa's Coral Reefs

Some of the oldest-living individuals in the world live near the coral reefs of Okinawa, Japan. While these people typically enjoy a simple diet rich in phytonutrients and free of fat-laden fast foods, this is not the only cause for their amazing longevity. The difference just may be in the water, which is naturally infused with marine-grade calcium from the nearby coral reefs. This marine-grade calcium, also called coral calcium, has been found to be easily digested and potent in its effects.

Coral calcium possesses some absolutely fascinating properties. For example, in addition to supporting bone density and health, coral calcium promotes heart health. It has been found to be incredibly effective in establishing and maintaining healthy blood pressure and blood lipid levels. It also helps assimilate vitamins and minerals from the foods you eat and the supplements you take. Coral calcium helps cleanse your kidneys, intestines, and liver by breaking down toxic heavy metals from environmental pollution. Its potent antioxidant activity protects your body from harmful free radical damage while also encouraging healthy oxygen levels. This dual action provides powerful help in fighting as well as preventing many types of cancer. Coral calcium also helps regulate blood sugar levels and even helps control digestive problems.

But one of coral calcium's most astonishing benefits is its effect on natural pH levels.

You have probably heard of pH balance, but have you ever considered its impact on your health? A good pH balance is extremely helpful in offsetting the typical Western diet that is high in fried foods, red meats, and simple starches.

It is also essential for the proper utilization of

nutrients, water, and oxygen. Your body's acidity content, or blood pH, needs to stay within a narrow range of between 7.35 and 7.45. Without this proper pH balance, your body is much more susceptible to disease. Diet, environmental toxins, and the aging process can tend to cause a poor pH balance, which in turn promotes the acceleration of free radical damage. Free radical damage contributes to virtually all chronic degenerative diseases, such as premature aging, stroke, and cancer. However, including coral calcium in your daily diet can help support the maintenance of a perfect pH balance as well as neutralize those dangerous free radicals, improving your body's overall health and its ability to fight degenerative diseases.

When you consume acidic elements and foods, components of your blood go to work neutralizing them. This neutralization process taps into your body's alkaline reserves, which are primarily calcium, magnesium, potassium, zinc, and sodium. Of all these minerals, though, calcium is the one mineral upon which your body relies most to ensure a properly balanced pH level. So, it certainly stands to reason that optimum absorption of this vital mineral is quite literally a matter of life or death. And that is where coral calcium's amazing natural ionic charge becomes a significant factor in maintaining good health.

Coral Calcium's Unique Ionic Charge

Calcium is found in abundance molecularly bound to our bones as well as in just about every one of our cells. When calcium is freed from this molecular bonding by a process called ionization, it combines with proteins and only *then* is it easily absorbed by the body. The ions contained in coral calcium possess a natural positive charge; this positive charge enables these ions to latch onto the negatively charged oxygen in vitamin D. This is called an ionic charge, and it is incredibly important to your health.

Think of it this way. If you hold two magnets, one in each hand, you will quickly discover that the positive pole of one magnet attracts the negative pole of the other. In much the same way, calcium has a positive charge and the oxygen in vitamin D has a negative charge, so they are attracted to each other.

When the ionized coral calcium latches onto the naturally occurring oxygen in vitamin D, it is then drawn into and through the intestinal wall and absorbed into the bloodstream. This natural ionic charge in coral calcium allows the body to absorb up to twenty times more essential calcium than any other form of calcium. In fact, coral calcium's amazing natural ionization allows for nearly one hundred percent bioavailability of this vital mineral.

Sango Coral is a Rich, Mineral-Laden Cornucopia of Good Health

Not only do the dazzlingly beautiful coral reefs of Okinawa offer the most absorbable form of calcium, they also provide the most perfectly complete complex of seventy-six essential minerals found anywhere in the world. These plant-based, organic, ocean minerals occur naturally in the algae that bonds with the coral. The result is nutrient-rich Sango coral, which is the only coral species out of the 2,500 species in the world that possesses the mineral content and proportions virtually identical to that of human bone. In fact, the composition of Sango coral is so close to human bone that surgeons around the world have successfully used it for bone grafts.

Highly absorbable calcium, seventy-six naturally occurring essential minerals, and a plethora of disease-fighting properties all combine to make Sango coral calcium superior to any other form of calcium. It simply is the most logical choice for improved good health and enhanced longevity.

In our next chapter, discover how some of nature's other amazing nutrients can actually maximize the absorption and benefits of good nutrition. So get ready for super-charged nutrition!

CHAPTER SEVEN
Kick Your Nutrient Absorption into Hyperdrive

Fulvic Acid Takes Great Nutrition to a Whole New Level

Doctors have known for years that in order to maintain optimum health, we need at least ninety nutrients. These nutrients include a minimum of fifty-nine minerals, sixteen vitamins, twelve amino acids, and three essential fatty acids. But eating great-tasting foods does not guarantee that your body absorbs or utilizes *any* of their vital nutrients. And when your body fails to absorb sufficient nutrients, you become extremely vulnerable to disease. That is where fulvic acid comes into the picture in a huge way. Scientists have found that fulvic acid is the one element in nature that facilitates the proper absorption of nutrients, making it something of a miracle molecule.

Interestingly, fulvic acid is not really a true acid at all. It is, however, the most powerfully effective nutrient delivery system found in nature. Fulvic acid has the ability to transport nutrients directly into your body's cellular structures. In fact, it can actually transport many times its weight in nutrients and elemental minerals. One single molecule of fulvic acid is capable of transporting as many as sixty or more minerals, vitamins, and trace elements into your body's cells. Fulvic acid also makes cell walls easier to penetrate so that nutrients can more easily enter the cell and waste can leave the cell more readily.

Unlike colloidal mineral molecules, which are too large to readily pass through cell walls, the presence of fulvic acid molecules actually makes minerals and vitamins much more absorbable. When fulvic acid is present, nutrients are dissolved into their most simple ionic form and then transported into and through tissue membranes and cell walls. Which means you will receive dramatically increased benefits from all nutrients, whatever the source, when fulvic acid is present.

Fulvic acid is a naturally occurring, supercharged, organic electrolyte that has an incredible ability to balance and energize biological properties. As such, it is quickly becoming recognized as one of the most critical factors in maintaining good health, even in the reversal and prevention of disease.

This "miracle molecule" also plays an important part in decreasing harmful acidic pH levels in your body by increasing the amount of beneficial oxygen in your blood. A lack of healthy blood oxygen is known to be a major contributor to acidic pH. And as we mentioned previously, an acidic pH level has been directly associated with practically every degenerative disease plaguing our world today, including cancer, cardiovascular disease, arthritis, osteoporosis, depression, kidney disorders, and a multitude of other health conditions.

Fulvic acid is one of the most powerful, natural free radical scavengers and antioxidants currently known. As we discussed in an earlier chapter, free radicals circulate throughout the body, injuring tissue and making cells susceptible to infections, diseases, and even cancer-causing mutations. Fulvic acid bonds to these free radicals and transforms them into organic, usable substances. If a cell is simply too damaged by these free radical molecules, then fulvic acid flushes the cell out of the body.

Fulvic acid also improves enzyme reactions in your body's cells by producing maximum stimulation of essential enzyme development. These enzymes serve as the life force behind vitamins and minerals. For example, a lack of sufficient digestive enzymes can cause stress in your digestive system, resulting in a malabsorption of nutrients.

Although fulvic acid is not an antibiotic in the technical sense of the word, its antibiotic-like effect is comparable to the power of penicillin in equally small amounts. And, unlike antibiotics, fulvic acid can be used indefinitely without creating an antibiotic resistant strain of disease, which is a common concern with prescription antibiotic drugs.

Several studies even indicate that fulvic acid extracts can effectively and safely kill the HIV virus. In fact, one pharmaceutical company has patented a fulvic-based drug that purifies blood for transfusions, killing the HIV virus without damaging healthy blood cells.

Indeed, the astounding health benefits of fulvic acid truly do qualify it as a "miracle molecule."

Sparkling Clean, Pure Water for Good Health and Nutrient Absorption

We all know that water is essential in maintaining life. It is estimated that the human body can subsist four to six weeks without food. However, living for just one week without water is nothing short of a miracle.

This makes sense when you consider that your body is made of around seventy-five percent water, your blood is more than eighty percent water, your brain is made up of over seventy-five percent water, and your liver is an astounding eighty-six percent water. With your body consisting of so much water, it is certainly obvious that it needs a constant flow of water to function at optimum efficiency.

Water is not only essential for life, it is also the system your body uses to transport nutrients. It is crucial for the proper absorption of vital nutrients that energize and activate every aspect and function of the solid matter in your body. Without the constant transportation of nutrients provided by water, your body's functions would quickly come to a halt.

Water is also an important factor in your body's biochemical reactions. For example, your body depends on water as part of the chemical reaction that allows proper digestion of protein and carbohydrates. This chemical reaction allows these nutrients to be quickly and efficiently absorbed.

So how much water should you drink daily? The amount varies from person to person, but according to many health professionals, men should consume around thirteen cups of water a day and women should consume at least nine cups of water daily in order to maintain proper hydration, nutrient absorption, and body system function.

However, it is important to realize that the *quality* of the water you drink is just as important as the *amount* of water that you drink. With the proliferation of pesticides, fertilizer run-off and industrial pollution, clean, pure drinking water has come to the forefront of consumer concerns—and rightfully so.

Between aging public supply water pipes and overwhelmed treatment plants, our nation's public water supplies have come under increasing scrutiny. For instance, ordinary tap water is known to contain an alarming number of chemicals that can cause irreparable damage to vital organs that act as natural filters—namely, the liver and kidneys.

More than 2,100 toxic chemicals have been found to currently exist in our nation's public water supplies. These chemicals include chloride—which was most notably used in World War II as a form of chemical warfare—as well as lead, arsenic, and a number of potential carcinogens.

It has also been revealed that an alarming array of prescription drugs is present in the drinking water of over forty-one million Americans. This is *after* the water has been supposedly purified at public water treatment plants. Some of the pharmaceuticals most commonly found in our drinking water are antibiotics, anti-convulsants, mood stabilizers, and estrogen. Trace levels of ibuprofen and acetaminophen are also present.

You might be even more surprised to learn that some drugs, including many popular cholesterol-lowering medications, tranquilizers, and anti-epileptic pharmaceuticals, actually resist traditional drinking water and wastewater treatment processes. There is also some evidence that by adding chlorine to water, which is a common practice in water treatment, some drugs become even more toxic.

Now consider the health effects of drinking such drug-laced water year after year. Recent studies have found that decades of low-level exposure to drugs, or random combinations of drugs, in our drinking water can have serious effects on human cells.

According to the Director of the Institute for Health and the Environment of the State University of New York at Albany, "We know we are being exposed to other people's drugs through our drinking water, and that can't be good."[8]

So while water is a vital element to support life, water contaminated with heavy metals, chemicals—including prescription drugs, and an array of other harmful toxins can have a decidedly detrimental effect on that life.

Reverse osmosis, also known as hyperfiltration, has become recognized as, quite simply, one of the most effective ways to ensure that the water we drink is free of contaminants and harmful bacteria. In fact, the process of reverse osmosis is used to produce water that meets the even most demanding specifications for purity.

This revolutionary process has the ability to remove particles as small as individual dissolved ions of contaminants as well as organic molecules from water by forcing the water through a microscopically thin membrane. As clean water is diffused through this membrane, a myriad of impurities is trapped in the membrane and flushed away.

Reverse osmosis effectively removes dissolved toxic chemicals and other impurities that can be harmful to your body's delicate systems. It also improves the taste of water, and reverse osmosis water will not produce the unsightly mineral buildup in kettles and coffee makers that regular tap water is notorious for. The process of reverse osmosis removes contaminants typically found in tap water, such as lead, copper, barium, chromium, mercury, sodium, cadmium, fluoride, nitrite, and nitrates. The result? Sparklingly clean, pure water.

Since water is so vitally crucial to our existence and good health, it only makes sense to answer your body's needs with the most pure water available. And reverse osmosis is the very best way to ensure that the water your body is utilizing is pure and free from harmful contaminants.

For this reason, it makes good sense to carefully screen the beverages, including bottled water, that you and your family consume. If they do not utilize reverse osmosis to ensure the highest level of filtration (be sure to check the label), you just don't know what contaminants may be lurking inside.

Likewise, only select nutritional supplements that feature reverse osmosis water as their base ingredient.

Micronization Vastly Increases Nutrient Absorption

Speaking of nutritional supplements, let's talk about micronization. The definition of micronization goes something like this: micronization is the process of reducing the average diameter of a solid material's particles. Usually, the term micronization is used when the particles produced are only a few micrometers in diameter. However, modern applications, which include the pharmaceutical and nutritional supplement industries, require average particle diameters in the scale of nanometers. So how do micronized particles affect the way your body absorbs nutrients?

When you ingest nutrients, whether in the form of fresh fruits and vegetables or in nutritional supplements, the size of the nutrient particles is of paramount importance. When molecules are too large to penetrate cellular membrane, your body simply cannot put them to maximum use. Micronization, however, breaks molecules down into nano-particles. This process enables the rapid absorption of natural compounds such as vitamins, minerals, and phytonutrients so that adequate concentrations appear in the blood. By decreasing the particle size to less than ten microns through a micronization process, both dissolution and bioavailability are immediately increased.

The long and short of it is this: the smaller the nutrient particles are, the more quickly and efficiently they are absorbed by the cells in your body, and the faster these nutrients are put to work to improve and maintain your good health.

Micronization actually increases the bio-availability of vital nutrients *and* enhances their absorption by as much as one hundred percent. With such astounding absorption rates as this, it just makes good sense to choose nutritional supplements that feature micronization technology.

CHAPTER EIGHT
The Sad State of Today's Foods

In the past seven chapters, you have learned how vitally important it is to have a diet filled with vitamins, minerals, phytonutrients, amino acids and other essential nutrients when it comes to bulletproofing your body against debilitating illnesses and maintaining good health. These life-giving nutrients are the fuel that your body was created to thrive upon.

However, in the ongoing efforts to feed a burgeoning world population, a dangerous health crisis has been created. Crops have, for more than one hundred years, been forced by using a chemical fertilizer that primarily contains the minerals nitrogen, phosphorus, and potassium. While these minerals are needed for crop growth, there are approximately seventy other essential minerals that have been systematically depleted from the soil. Plants will grow under these deficient conditions, but they are severely lacking in nutrients required for human sustenance. The sad truth is that by neglecting to replenish these missing minerals for so many years, our soil has become exhausted and depleted of essential nutrients.

Vitamins and minerals act as co-factors for each other. This means that each vitamin depends on a specific mineral to make it work and vice versa. Without the proper co-factors in the proper ratios, neither vitamins nor minerals can be effective. This health danger was recognized at least seventy years ago, when Document #264 was presented to the 74th Congress of the United States Senate in 1936. The basic thrust of this document was that foods being grown in millions of acres of American soil no longer contained enough of certain vital minerals, and that this mineral depletion was starving the population—no matter how much of these foods were consumed. Imagine how much more severe this problem has become all these years later as the ground has continued to be stripped of nutrients.

It is a tragic fact that you can no longer derive all of the crucial nutrients your body needs exclusively from today's fruits, vegetables, and grains, no matter how healthy your diet. Yes, plants do manufacture vitamins, but they cannot manufacture minerals. And vitamins can only be utilized properly if minerals are present in the proper ratios. If your daily diet does not provide all the needed essential nutrients, the chemical reactions that make vitamins useable cannot take place. This means that you can eat the healthiest foods available and still not receive the benefit of the vitamins in that food—simply because without minerals, vitamins are largely ineffective.

Considering the fact that there are approximately seventy to eighty-four essential minerals that your body must have to function properly and only three of these minerals are regularly replenished in our soil, it is not such a huge leap to recognize that, while our stomachs may be full, our bodies are starving. As a society, we are becoming more and more nutritionally deficient with each passing day. With such a serious lack of nutrients, your body has very little chance of maintaining the vibrantly good health it was created to enjoy.

Recognizing this serious nutritional crisis, the *Journal of the American Medical Association* published an article in 2002 addressing the use of vitamin and mineral supplements and the prevention of chronic disease. After reviewing the body of evidence, researchers advised their medical colleagues that the use of vitamin/mineral supplements was a prudent intervention in the fight against many chronic, degenerative diseases. The article concluded with the recommendation that Americans should include a vitamin/ mineral supplement in their daily diet.

The bottom line is that even in a perfect world of nine daily servings of fresh fruits and vegetables and a diet free of fast foods, our bodies often simply need more. To get the optimum nutrition that will sustain our bodies and support vibrantly good health, we should each include a high-quality vitamin/mineral supplement.

So For Good Health, Start with a Strong Foundation

If your lifestyle includes a healthy diet filled with plenty of fresh fruits and vegetables, do you *really* need to take a vitamin/mineral supplement? Not so very long ago, most experts would have probably said that no, it was not necessary.

However, today the vast majority of those same experts would likely say that including a high-quality daily nutritional supplement makes sense for most adults.

In fact, the Harvard School of Public Health

has stated, "Intake of several vitamins above the minimum daily requirement may help prevent heart disease, cancer, osteoporosis, and other chronic diseases."[9]

So what should you look for when choosing the best vitamin/mineral supplement for you and your family? Three categories of nutrients that your body needs should be present in any nutritional supplement you consider. These three categories are:

Vitamins, minerals, and trace minerals

Fruits, vegetables, and fulvic acid

Coral calcium, antioxidants, and amino acids

These three categories form the strongest nutritional foundation possible for your good health and the good health of your family.

As we have discussed throughout this book, proper nutrition with a daily supply of essential vitamins, minerals, trace minerals, and other nutrients affects longevity, disease prevention, growth and development, emotional health, intelligence, quality of life, and behavior.

Whether you are four or 104, your body needs these nutrients every day in order to thrive.

Now let's talk about the form of your nutritional supplements. Tablets versus capsules, capsules versus liquid. Which is the best choice? You may be surprised to learn that your body is only able to absorb about ten to twenty percent of the nutrients contained in tablet supplements. The reason is simple—matter can only remain in your stomach for a very limited amount of time. Inside your stomach, natural digestive acids go to work breaking down the food, tablets, or capsules that you have ingested. What does not break down quickly is simply flushed from your body via natural elimination. Pressed tablets are very slow to dissolve, with the majority of their beneficial nutrients simply passing out of your body unused. Capsules are certainly more easily absorbed than tablets, but by far your best choice is a liquid nutritional supplement.

When in a liquid form, nutritional supplements are immediately absorbed by your body's cellular structures with little or no digestion process. This ensures maximum absorption, quite nearly one hundred percent, of the vital nutrients your body requires to maintain glowing good health.

CHAPTER NINE
Don't Wait For A Health Crisis
—Become Proactive, Not Reactive

By design, prescription drugs are reactive in nature. They are developed to address specific illnesses or, more often, specific *symptoms* of illnesses.

No one takes a statin drug such as Crestor before he or she is diagnosed with high cholesterol. No one takes harsh anti-inflammatory medications like Vioxx before suffering the debilitating pain of inflamed joints or arthritis. These drugs, along with the vast majority of other prescription medications, are reactive because they only offer treatment *after* a health issue has manifested. And, as described earlier, such prescriptive medications are all too often fraught with harmful, even fatal, side effects.

It is important to understand that disease begins on a cellular level long before symptoms of that illness appear. Your body has little chance of maintaining good health year after year if it is consistently deprived of the tools it needs to function properly.

Although it seems that many diseases appear suddenly, the sad truth is they are usually the result of years of deficiency that could have easily been reversed through a lifestyle of proper diet, exercise and nutritional supplementation.

The very best time to begin incorporating a healthy diet, exercise, and quality nutritional supplements into your lifestyle is *before* you experience a health crisis. This is a key step toward establishing a lifestyle of wellness, not sickness.

Taking care of our bodies should be a natural part of any lifestyle; however, the truth is that many times it takes a crisis to stir us into taking action.

Years of improper diet without the benefit of nutritional supplementation, lack of exercise and environmental pollution can eventually add up to serious health challenges. Even though it often takes years of neglect for our bodies to degenerate to the point that symptoms appear, the good news is that, many times, lifestyle changes can result in a rapid return to good health.

Each person's body responds to the benefits of optimum nutrition differently. Some experience nearly immediate results, while others notice subtle changes with a gradual progress toward renewed health.

The bottom line is this—regardless of your current state of health, embracing a lifestyle of proper nutrition and exercise is absolutely essential for your body to sustain the kind of thriving good health it was created to enjoy.

Imagine a Life Free From Illness and Debilitating Disease...a Life Filled With Energy, Vitality, and Amazing Longevity

This kind of energetic, healthy life is what our bodies were designed for, but poor nutritional choices, a sedentary lifestyle, and an overabundance of chemically based pharmaceuticals have stolen it from all of us. So become proactive and take charge of your health and your life today. Become an educated consumer when it comes to what you put into your body and the bodies of your family.

Before you take another drug, whether over-the-counter or prescription, find out what its side effects are. Remember, all prescription drugs—without exception—have side effects. Ask your doctor questions about known adverse effects of the prescription he or she is about to write for you.

Make the decision to include some form of exercise in your family's daily routine—every day. You do not necessarily need a gym membership to get in shape, just a little creativity and determination.

Take your family for a walk, go roller skating or biking, or even take up dancing. Anything that gets your body moving and your heart pumping is going to melt away unwanted pounds, increase your energy level, and sharply reduce your susceptibility to disease.

Keep your meals as close to the earth as possible, meaning choose fresh foods over preservative-laden, pre-processed foods. And stay far away from fast food restaurants! Sure, they're convenient, but is convenience really worth the extra pounds and associated poor health?

Remember to start each day with a high-quality liquid nutritional supplement that contains the vitamins, minerals, amino acids and other nutrients discussed in this book. This, along with exercise and a diet free of dangerous preservatives and chemically altered fats, will go a long way toward bulletproofing your body against a life tragically cut short by the effects of obesity and disease.

When it comes to resolving and even preventing many of the debilitating diseases that plague today's society, you do have a choice. Prescription drugs are not the "end all, be all" that drug companies would like you to believe.

Instead, look to the wisdom and wealth of *nature's* medicine chest.

ENDNOTES

Chapter One: The Billion-Dollar Business of Illness

NaturalNews.com. 22 February 2007; <http://www.naturalnews.com/021635.html>

Journal American Medical Association. 26 July 26 2000; 284(4):483–5

<http://jama.ama-assn.org/cgi/content/abstract/296/13/1619>

Journal American Medical Association. Vol 284; 26 July 2000

Chapter Four: Nature's Medicine Chest

Journal of Nutrition. 2006; 136:810S-812S;

March 2006 The American Society for Nutrition <http://jn.nutrition.org/cgi/content/full/136/3/810S>

University of Maryland Medical Center; <http://www.umm.edu/altmed/articles/garlic-000245.htm>

Chapter Five: The ABC's of Nutritional Vitamins and Minerals

Selenium and Prostate Cancer. The Health Report; 7 December 1998; <http://www.abc.net.au/rn/talks/8.30/helthrpt/stories/s17802.htm>

Ishida, B.K., Turner, C., Chapman, M.H., MCKeon, T.A. 2004; Fatty acids and carotenoid composition in gas (momordica cochinchinensis spreng) fruit. Journal of Agricultural and Food Chemistry, Vol 52, p. 274279.

Chapter Seven: Kick Your Nutrient Absorption into Hyperdrive

AP Probe Finds Drugs In Drinking Water; Yahoo! News; 09 March 2008; http://news. yahoo.com/s/ap/20080309/ap_on_re_us/ pharmawater_i&printer=1>

Chapter Eight: The Sad State of Today's Foods

Harvard School of Public Health. 2007; <http://www.hsph.harvard.edu/nutrition-source/vitamins.html>

BIBLIOGRAPHY

Prescription Drug Deaths Skyrocket 60 Percent
Over Five Years As Americans Swallow More
Pills; NaturalNews.com; viewed 22 February 2007 - http://www.naturalnews.com/
z021635.html

Hormone Replacement Therapy for the Prevention of Chronic Conditions in Postmeno-
pausal Women; U.S. Preventative Services
Task Force; May 2005; viewed 18 February
2007 - <http://www.ahrq.gov/clinic/uspstf/
uspspmho.htm>

Decrease in Breast Cancer Rates Related to

Reduction in Use of Hormone Replacement Therapy; National Institutes of Health NIH News; 18 April 2007; viewed 25 June 2007 - <http://www.nih.gov/news/pr/apr2007/nci-18a.htm>

WIH Finds No Heart Disease Benefit, Increased Stroke Risk With Estrogen Alone; National Institutes of Health NIH News; 13 April 2004; viewed 25 June 2007 - <http://www.nhlbi.nih.gov/new/press/04-04-13.htm>

U.S. Preventative Services Task Force Evidence Syntheses, Hormone Replacement Therapy and Breast Cancer Systematic Evidence Review; viewed 5 December 2007 - <http://www.ncbi.nlm.nih.gov/books/bv.fcgi?rid=hstat3.chapter.27252>

Women's Health Initiative; 10 October 2007; viewed 15 November 2007 - <http://www.nhlbi.nih.gov/whi>

Doctors May Be Third Leading Cause of Death;

Chattanooga Health.com; 15 March 2000; viewed 12 November 2007 - http://www.chattanoogahealth.com/Articles/2135/1/Doctors_May_Be_Third_Leading_Cause_of_Death.aspx

Unintentional Poisoning Deaths–United States, 1999–2004; CDC; 56(05);93–96; 9 February 2007

Statistics Prove Prescription Drugs Are 16,400% More Deadly Than Terrorists; NewsTarget.com; 5 July 2005; viewed 5 November 2007 - http://newstarget.com/z009278.html

To Err Is Human–Building a Safer Health System; Institute of Medicine; 2000; viewed 2 April 2007 - <http://www.nap.edu/openbook.php?isbn=0309068371>

75 Percent Of Americans Overweight By 2015; MSNBC; 19 July 2007; viewed 15 November 2007 - http://msnbc.com/id/19845784/from/ET

Obesity Tied To Increased Risk For Dozens Of Conditions; 22 November 2004; viewed 22 February 2007 - <http://www.eurekalert.org/pub_releases/2004–11/cfta-ott111904.php>

Just Say No to Prescription Drugs; Natural-News.com; 4 December 2007; viewed 19 December 2007 - <http://www.naturalnews.com/z022322.html>

New Online Consumer Health Guide Reveals Nutritional Deficiencies Caused By Prescription Drugs; Natural News.com; 10 September 2007; viewed 3 November 2007 - <http://naturalnews.com/z022022.html>

National Osteoporosis Foundation; viewed 22 January 2008 - < http://www.nof.org>

Calcium Absorption from the Ingestion of Coral-Derived Calcium by Humans; J Nut. Sci Vit, lmino; J 999, 45, 509–517; Higashi Sapporo Hospital, Sapporo 003–8585, Japan

1 Formerly, Tokyo University of Agriculture, Ichikawa 272–0035, Japan 3 Division of Applied Food Research, The National Institute of Health and Nutrition, Tokyo 162–8636, Japan

Tainted Drinking Water Kept Under Wraps; Associated Press; 09 March 2008; viewed 09 March 2008 - http://www.msnbc.msn.com/id/23504373/

AP Probe Finds Drugs In Drinking Water; Yahoo! News; 09 March 2008; viewed 09 March 2008 - http://news.yahoo.com/s/ap/20080309/ap_on_re_us/pharmawater_i&printer=1>

ABOUT THE AUTHORS

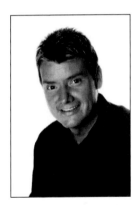

Mark A. Stevens—a successful businessman, noted author, and motivational speaker—is passionate about shining a bright spotlight on the phenomenal health benefits of what he calls "nature's medicine chest." As a child, Mark watched helplessly as his chronically ill mother sought relief from debilitating health issues—which often included handfuls of new prescriptions, each of which added to a cascading tide of adverse side affects. The memory of feeling powerless to help someone he dearly loved became the driving force in his life mission to help people enjoy fruitful lives, filled with good health, energy, and vitality. This fervent determination led him to seek out and establish lasting relationships with a number of respected medical professionals and nutrition experts, including nutritional chemists. Through these relationships, Mark has gleaned a deep understanding of the life-enriching benefits of natural nutrition. His creed and life principle is that, together, we can make the world a better, healthier place . . . one life at a time.

Christine A. Jones is a writer and editor residing with her family in Oklahoma. As Christine began investigating our nation's alarming rise in health problems, she found that the secret to good health and longevity is, oftentimes, completely within our grasp through well-informed nutritional and lifestyle choices. This discovery has fueled a passionate mission to educate the public regarding the dangers of poor nutritional choices and sedentary lifestyles.